THE SECRET LIFE OF COFFEE

A caffeine-fueled memoir

A caffeine-fueled memoir that will make you laugh, cry, and maybe even jolt you out of your seat!

Introduction: Coffee: A Love Story

Part 1: A Beginner's Buzz

Chapter 1: Falling for Coffee

Chapter 2: Coffeehouse Culture

Chapter 3: From Sip to Savor: Tasting Coffee

Part 2: A World of Beans

Chapter 4: The Global Coffee Trade

INTRODUCTION

COFFEE : A LOVE STORY

Coffee, ah. The enchanted potion that cheers up our days and unites people. For me, coffee has always represented a love story more than just a beverage. A love story that started long ago and is still standing strong. Sure, it's not a real relationship, but at least I don't have to worry about my coffee ever cheating on me.

My first cup of coffee is still fresh in my mind. I was a youngster at the time, and I was always entranced by the potent coffee aroma that permeated the air each morning. So I decided to try it one day. When I took the first sip, I still feel a warm sensation spreading throughout my body. I felt something I had never felt before, and I immediately realized I had found something wonderful.

Coffee became a fixture in my life as I grew older, joined by friends. I learned to enjoy coffee flavors, such as how an espresso shot is strong and robust or a creamy latte is sweet and soothing.

But I didn't really discover how much I loved coffee until I started traveling. I learned new ways to drink coffee in many places around the world. In Italy, I discovered how to appreciate the art of sipping a perfectly prepared espresso while seated at a bar. I first experienced the pleasure of drinking strong, black coffee while relaxing in a café and observing daily life in Turkey. Then I sampled coffee in its purest form, straight from the source, in Ethiopia. I've become more social because of my coffee love. I've sat across from friends and loved ones and shared countless cups of coffee while we spoke over a warm mug of coffee. Over coffee, I've had thoughtful discussions and fun exchanges and laughter.

Moreover, there are coffee cafes. I've always found refuge in these warm, welcoming places, where I can shut off the outside world and lose myself in a book or my thoughts. I've spent endless hours in coffee shops trying out various blends, observing people, and socializing. My affection for coffee hasn't always been apparent, though. I've had enough of subpar cups of coffee, as well as the dreaded caffeine jitters. Yet even then, I couldn't help but like coffee. I wouldn't want it any other way; it's fundamental to me.

Now that I'm sitting here with a warm cup of coffee, I can't help but think back on my romance with this wonderful potion. There have been highs and lows along the way, but coffee has always been there for me. And I'm confident that wherever life takes me, I'll always have a warm coffee mug to cheer me up and keep me grounded. My relationship with coffee has been long and beautiful. The plot of this narrative is still being developed, and I'm eager to find out where it will lead. Because, at its core, coffee is a way of life rather than a beverage. And I'm honored to participate.

PART 1

A BEGINNER'S BUZZ

CHAPTER 1 : FALLING FOR COFFEE

As I walk into my favorite coffee shop, the aroma of freshly brewed coffee greets me, and my mouth waters with anticipation. The sound of beans being ground, the hiss of steam, and the chatter of fellow coffee lovers all combine to create a warm and inviting atmosphere. I can't help but smile as I take it all in. As I take it all in, I remember that I forgot to put on pants!

I remember when I first fell for coffee. It was during my freshman year of college, and I struggled to stay awake during long study sessions. I had always been a tea drinker, but it just wasn't cutting it anymore. So, one day, I decided to try coffee, and I was hooked from the first sip. I even had to get a bigger backpack to carry around my coffee thermos!

At first, I was hesitant to explore the world of coffee beyond the basic drip coffee in the dining hall. But as I experimented with different coffee types, I discovered a whole new world of flavors and aromas. I learned about the different roasts, brewing methods, and even the beans' origin. It was like discovering an exciting hobby, and I couldn't get enough.

Before long, I became a regular at my local coffee shop, and the baristas knew me by name. I loved trying out their daily specials, which often featured exotic flavors and unique brewing methods. I even experimented with making my own coffee at home, investing in a quality grinder and French press.

But it wasn't just the coffee taste that drew me in. It was the ritual of it all. The process of grinding the beans, heating the water, and patiently waiting for the coffee to brew became a peaceful and meditative part of my morning routine. It was a moment of calm before the day's chaos began.

Now, years later, I can confidently say that I have fallen for coffee. It's become a part of who I am, a daily ritual that brings me joy and comfort. And while I know there are many other beverages out there to explore, I'll always have a special place in my heart (and my taste buds) for my favorite cup of coffee.

As I continued to explore the world of coffee, I became more interested in the culture and history behind it. I learned about coffee's origins, tracing them back to Ethiopia and the legend of Kaldi and his dancing goats. I read about coffee's spread throughout the Middle East, Europe, and eventually the Americas, and the impact it had on global trade and culture.

I also discovered the art of latte art, where baristas use steamed milk to create intricate designs on the surface of a latte. I was amazed by the skill and creativity of these artists and even tried my hand at it a few times (with mixed results).

But it wasn't just the coffee itself that drew me in. It was the social aspect of it all. Meeting up with friends for a cup of coffee became a regular occurrence. We often spend hours chatting and catching up over a latte or cappuccino.

I also loved visiting quaint coffee shops and discovering their unique atmosphere and personality. Some were cozy and rustic, with exposed brick walls and wooden tables, while others were sleek and modern, with minimalist decor and high-tech brewing equipment. Each one had its own vibe and charm, and I loved experiencing them all.

As my love for coffee grew, I appreciated its health benefits. Research has shown that moderate coffee consumption can reduce the risk of several chronic diseases, including type 2 diabetes, liver disease, and certain types of cancer. It can also improve cognitive function and boost mood and energy levels.

Of course, like anything, coffee has downsides. We Too much caffeine can lead to jitters, anxiety, and disrupted sleep patterns. And some people may experience digestive issues or other negative side effects.

But for me, coffee's benefits far outweigh the risks. It's a daily pleasure I look forward to, a moment of comfort and indulgence in an otherwise busy and stressful world. And as long as there are new beans to try, creative brewing methods to experiment with, and new coffee shops to visit, I know my love for coffee will continue to grow.

CHAPTER 2: COFFEE HOUSE CULTURE

Upon entering my favorite coffee shop, the familiar scent of freshly brewed coffee and the sound of people chatting and laughing fill the air. I take a deep breath and feel comfort wash over me. For me, this is not just a place to grab a caffeine fix. Instead, it is a haven where I can escape the chaos of the outside world and indulge in a moment of "me time".

Coffee house culture has always fascinated me. From the first coffee houses in 16th century Constantinople to the trendy cafes of modern-day cities, coffee houses have played a crucial role in shaping culture and society. And for me, there is something magical about sipping a hot cup of coffee in others' company.

One of the things I love most about coffee house culture is the sense of community it creates. Coffee shops are often gathering places where people from all walks of life come together to share coffee and conversation. It's not uncommon to strike up a conversation with a stranger, exchange book recommendations or share a laugh over a funny meme.

In addition to being social hubs, coffee shops also serve as creative spaces for artists, writers, and entrepreneurs. Coffee houses offer free Wi-Fi and a quiet atmosphere, making them the most appropriate spot to work on a project or brainstorm ideas. I've lost count of the number of times I've seen someone scribbling in a notebook or typing away on a laptop at a nearby table.

But coffee house culture is not just about the social aspect - it's also about the coffee itself. Coffee is a complex and nuanced beverage, with endless variations in flavor, aroma, and texture. From the fruity notes of a light roast to the smoky richness of a dark roast, there is something for everyone. And with the rise of specialty coffee shops, consumers have access to a wider variety of beans and brewing methods than ever before.

Of course, coffee house culture has downsides. The cost of a daily coffee habit can add up quickly, and caffeine can have negative effects on health. And not all coffee shops are created equal - some may be crowded and noisy, while others may lack the atmosphere or quality of coffee I seek.

But for me, coffee house culture's positives far outweigh the negatives. Whether I'm catching up with a friend over a latte or settling in with my favorite book and a pour-over, the coffee shop is a place where I can relax, recharge, and connect with others. It's a ritual I look forward to every day. It will continue to be a part of my life for a long time to come, and I'm sure I'll treasure it.

CHAPTER 3: FROM SIP TO SAVOR: TASTING COFFEE

As someone who takes coffee a lot, I have come to appreciate the beauty and complexity of this beloved beverage. Each cup of coffee is an unforgettable experience, filled with subtle nuances and intricate flavors that can transport me to different parts of the world and awaken my senses.

When I enter a coffee shop, I'm immediately drawn to the rich and inviting aroma of freshly brewed coffee. It's a scent I know and love, one that signals a new adventure.

As I approach the counter, I already know what I want - a bold and flavorful cup of coffee that will kickstart my day. I ask the barista for their recommendation, eager to try something new and exciting.

When my coffee is ready, I admire its deep and rich color,

admiring the way the light reflects off the liquid surface. I inhale deeply, savoring the aroma of freshly brewed coffee and the complex notes of chocolate, citrus, and caramel.

With the first sip, I'm transported to a different world. The coffee flavor is bold and invigorating, filling me with energy and vitality. I let the liquid roll over my tongue, savoring the different flavors and sensations as they dance across my palate.

As I drink, I become more attuned to coffee nuances. I can taste the different layers of flavor, from the bright and tangy acidity to the deep and earthy undertones. With each sip, I feel more connected to the world around me, more alive and awake.

For me, drinking coffee is not just about getting a caffeine boost - it's a ritual, a way to connect with the world and experience new flavors and sensations. With each cup of coffee, I'm reminded of the beauty and complexity of life. I'm grateful for the opportunity to savor each moment. I'm also grateful for the opportunity to use the restroom after drinking each cup!

PART 2

A WORLD OF BEANS

CHAPTER 4: THE GLOBAL COFFEE TRADE

I have always been fascinated by the global coffee trade. The journey each coffee bean takes from its origin to my cup is intricate and intriguing.

Global coffee trade is a massive industry that involves farmers, traders, roasters, and retailers. Coffee beans are grown in tropical regions around the world, including Latin America, Africa, and Asia. Each region produces coffee beans with unique flavors and characteristics, depending on the climate, soil, and growing conditions.

As I sip my morning coffee, I can't help but think about the journey this coffee bean has taken. It likely began its journey on a small coffee farm in Colombia. It was carefully picked by hand and then processed to remove the outer layers of the bean. The process of removing the outer layers can be done in different ways, depending on the farm's location and tradition. In some places, the beans are washed with water to wash away the mucilage. In others they are left to dry on raised beds or patios until the outer layer becomes brittle and can be eliminated through mechanical or manual hulling. From there, the green coffee beans were shipped to a coffee trader, who evaluated its quality and sold it to a roaster.

Coffee traders play a crucial role in the coffee supply chain. They source beans directly from farmers or cooperatives, and sell them to roasters. In many cases, coffee traders also act as quality controllers, ensuring that coffee beans meet the necessary standards for flavor, aroma, and appearance. These standards are set by organizations like the Specialty Coffee Association, which provides a global framework for quality control and sustainability practices.

Once the coffee beans arrive at the roaster's facility, they are roasted to perfection, bringing out their unique flavors and aromas. Roasting is an art form that requires skill, precision, and knowledge. Roasters carefully monitor the roast temperature and time to achieve the desired flavor profile. They also use their expertise to blend different types of coffee beans to create signature blends that appeal to their customers.

After roasting, coffee beans are packaged and shipped to retailers and coffee shops around the world. In recent years, there has been a growing trend towards direct trade, where coffee roasters source their beans directly from farmers or cooperatives. This trade model allows for enhanced transparency and fair prices for farmers.

But the journey doesn't end there. Once the coffee beans arrive at their final destination, they are brewed into a delicious cup of coffee by skilled baristas who understand the art of coffee-making. Coffee preparation can vary greatly depending on the method and preferences of the coffee shop or individual. Some prefer espresso machines, while others use the pour-over or French press methods. Baristas also play a vital role in educating customers about the origins and flavor profiles of different types of coffee. They also teach them how to brew them at home.

As I take another sip of my coffee, I am grateful for the many people and processes that have come together to create this delicious cup of coffee. Global coffee trade is deeply rooted in tradition and community. Coffee has been a part of human culture for centuries, and coffee-making has been passed down from generation to generation. It is an industry that connects people from different parts of the world, creating a sense of shared culture and appreciation for the simple pleasures of life.

Despite its complexity, the global coffee trade faces many challenges. Climate change, disease outbreaks, and labor rights are all issues that affect the sustainability of the coffee industry. As consumers, we can make a positive impact by supporting ethical and sustainable practices in the coffee supply chain.

CHAPTER 5

ROASTING : THE ART OF TURNING GREEN BEANS BROWN

As a coffee enthusiast, I have always been fascinated by roasting. The art of turning green coffee beans into rich, aromatic brown beans is a true testament to coffee roasters' skill and expertise.

Roasting involves heating green coffee beans until they reach a specific temperature and color. The roasting process transforms the chemical and physical properties of the coffee bean. This results in distinct flavors and aromas associated with different coffee types.

Roasting is a delicate process that requires precision and attention to detail. Coffee roasters carefully monitor the beans' temperature and adjust the drying time to achieve the desired flavor profile. The temperature of the roasting machine, the airflow, and the roasting time are all factors that influence the final flavor and aroma of the coffee.

One of the most fascinating aspects of roasting is the science behind it. During the roasting process, coffee beans undergo complex chemical reactions. The heat causes the sugars and acids in coffee beans to break down and form new compounds, creating unique flavors and aromas.

The roasting process can vary depending on the type of coffee bean and the desired flavor profile. For example, lighter roasts are typically roasted for a shorter amount of time and at lower temperatures, resulting in a brighter, more acidic flavor. Dark roasts, on the other hand, are roasted for longer periods at higher temperatures. This results in a bold, full-bodied flavor with a smoky or chocolaty undertone.

Roasting is truly an art form, and the finest coffee roasters take pride in their craft. They spend years honing their skills, experimenting with different roasting techniques, and constantly improving coffee quality. A skilled coffee roaster knows how to bring out the unique flavors and aromas of each coffee bean, creating a truly exceptional cup of coffee.

As a coffee lover, I appreciate the dedication and work and dedication into the roasting process. The art of roasting is a testament to human ingenuity and creativity. It is an industry that is constantly evolving, with advancing techniques and technologies to improve coffee quality and sustainability.

The next time you enjoy a delicious cup of coffee, appreciate roasting art. From the careful selection of green coffee beans to the precise monitoring of the roasting process, every step is a testament to the coffee roaster's skill and dedication. It is a process that has been refined over centuries, and continues to inspire and delight coffee lovers around the world.

CHAPTER 6

BREWING TECHNIQUES: FINDING YOUR PERFECT CUP

As a coffee lover, I have always sought the perfect cup of coffee. And I have discovered that the key to that perfect cup lies in the brewing technique.

There are countless brewing methods out there, each with its own unique characteristics and advantages. Whether you prefer the smooth, rich taste of a French press or the bold, robust flavor of a pour-over, there is a brewing method out there that is right for you.

One of the most significant factors in brewing an excellent cup of coffee is the grind. The size and consistency of the coffee grounds can have a significant impact on the flavor and aroma of the final product. A coarse grind is ideal for French press methods, while a finer grind is better suited to espresso.

Another key factor is the water temperature. Water that is too hot can scorch the coffee, while water that is too cold can cause a weak, insipid cup. Ideally, the water temperature should be between 195 and 205 degrees Fahrenheit for most brewing methods.

Brewing time is also crucial to the perfect cup. For example, a French press should be steeped for 3-4 minutes, while a pour-over should be brewed for 2-3 minutes.

One of my favorite brewing methods is the pour-over. It is a simple, yet elegant technique that allows precise control over the brewing process. The key is to slowly pour hot water over the coffee grounds. This allows the water to fully saturate the beans and extract the desired flavors and aromas.

I have found that experimenting with different brewing methods and techniques is the most convenient way to find my perfect cup of coffee. Whether it's trying another brewing method, tweaking the grind size, or adjusting the water temperature, every small change can have a significant impact on the final product.

But the most defining factor in brewing an excellent cup of coffee is the bean quality. No matter how skilled the brewing technique, if the beans are poor, the final product will be lackluster. That's why I always choose high-quality, freshly roasted coffee beans.

Brewing the perfect cup of coffee is both an art and a science. It requires skill, patience, and willingness to experiment. But the result is a delicious, aromatic cup of coffee that brightens any morning.

So, whether you prefer a bold, robust coffee or a smooth, delicate cup, experiment with different brewing techniques. You will find the method that works best for you. With a little practice and experimentation, you too can achieve the perfect cup of coffee.

PART 3

A DAY IN THE LIFE OF A COFFEE ADDICT

CHAPTER 7 : A MORNING RITUAL

I wake up every morning to the sound of my alarm clock, the shrill beeps breaking the stillness of the early hours. Even before my eyes open, I know what I'm craving. A hot, strong cup of coffee. My day doesn't begin until I complete my morning ritual.

I shuffle my feet as I walk to the kitchen, still half asleep. I turn on the coffee machine and wait for it to warm up. As I wait, I stretch my arms and legs, trying to shake off the grogginess of the night before. Finally, the coffee machine is ready, and I carefully measure out the appropriate amount of coffee grounds. I grind the beans to a fine consistency and add them to the filter.

As the coffee brews, the aroma fills the kitchen. It's a smell that brings me comfort and sets the tone for the day ahead. I love the scent of freshly brewed coffee. Its rich aroma and warmth fill my senses. It's a sign of the day's beginning, an indication that things are about to start.

I pour myself a cup and take my first sip. The hot liquid awakens my senses, and I feel more alert than a few minutes ago. It's as if a switch has been flipped and my mind is suddenly more awake and ready to face the day. There's something about that first sip of coffee that's magical.

I take my coffee to my favorite spot in the house, a cozy corner with a view of the outdoors. I sit in my chair, and with each sip, I feel more energized. As I sip, I see the view outside, the sun slowly rising above the horizon. I also hear the gentle breeze rustling the trees' leaves. It's peaceful and serene, the happiest way to start my day.

As I finish my cup, I feel a sense of calm. My morning ritual has become a vital part of my day, providing a moment of tranquility before the hustle and bustle of work and daily life. It's a small moment of mindfulness in a hectic and overwhelming world.

But my morning coffee isn't just about caffeine. It's about ritual, the routine. It's a way to start my day on the right foot, to set a positive tone for what's to come. It's a small act of self-care, a reminder that I deserve a few moments of peace and quiet each day.

Without my morning ritual, my day wouldn't be the same. It's the most ideal way to kick off my day, and I wouldn't have it any other way. As I finish my coffee and start my day, I know that no matter what comes my way, I'll face it with a bit more energy and positivity.

My morning ritual has become a tradition, an unspoken agreement between myself and the universe that this is how my day will start. It's not just a cup of coffee, but a connection to something bigger. It's a symbol of the start of another day and all of the possibilities that come with it.

As the morning light fills my home, I take a deep breath and remind myself that no matter what comes my way, I'm always prepared. Ready to face the day, ready to take on the challenges, and ready to embrace the opportunities that come with it. And it all starts with that first coffee sip in the morning.

CHAPTER 8: COFFEE ON THE GO

A good day doesn't start until I have my cup of coffee. But, with a busy schedule and a never-ending to-do list, I can't always sit down and enjoy a cup of coffee at home. That's why I've mastered coffee on the go. As the old saying goes, "If you can't beat the coffee-drinking habits, join them!"

My morning routine starts with a quick shower and getting dressed for the day ahead. As I grab my bag and rush out the door, I grab my travel mug filled with my favorite coffee blend. The smell of freshly brewed coffee fills my senses as I take my first sip, and I know it's going to be a good day.

As I walk to work, the city comes alive around me. People rush past me, cars honk, and the city sounds are all around. But, with my coffee in hand, I feel calm and relaxed. It's my tranquil oasis in the city chaos.

When I reach my office, I savor the last few sips of my coffee before the day's work begins. It's my moment of calm before the storm. I feel energized and ready to take on whatever challenges the day has in store for me.

But, my love of coffee doesn't stop there. As the day progresses, I often need a caffeine boost. That's when I turn to my trusty travel mug. Whether I'm running from one meeting to the next or trying to finish a project before a deadline, a quick sip of coffee keeps me on track.

In fact, my travel mug has become my constant companion, my partner in crime. It's always by my side, helping me power through the day, no matter how busy or stressful it may be. And, in those moments when I need a break from the hustle and bustle, I take a few minutes to enjoy a few sips of my coffee. I take in the world around me.

Whether I'm on the go or sitting at my desk, coffee is essential to my day. It's a source of comfort, a reminder of home, and a way to keep my mind sharp and my body energized. And, with my trusty travel mug in hand, I know I can take on anything that comes my way.

So, whether I'm rushing to a meeting, running errands, or simply enjoying the sights and sounds of the city, my coffee is always with me. This is a constant reminder that life is better with caffeine. And, as I take my last sip of the day, I know that tomorrow will be another day. This day will be full of endless possibilities and opportunities to enjoy my beloved coffee on the go.

CHAPTER 9: COFFEE AT WORK

I can't imagine working without my trusty cup of Joe. Whether it's a busy day full of meetings and deadlines or a slow day with little to do, my coffee keeps me focused and energized.

My morning routine starts with a quick stop at the coffee machine in the break room. The sound of the machine brewing my coffee is like music to my ears, and the aroma of freshly brewed coffee fills the air. I carefully choose my blend, pour it into my favorite mug, and add a splash of creamer.

As I settle into my workday, coffee is my constant companion. It sits at my desk, steaming and beckoning me with every sip. It's a source of comfort and motivation, reminding me that I can conquer any task that comes my way.

And, on those particularly long and challenging days, my coworkers know that the most effective way to cheer me up is to offer me a cup of coffee. It's like a little encouragement, a reminder that I'm not alone in my struggles.

But, my love of coffee isn't just about the caffeine boost. It's also about coffee's social aspect at work. It's a way to connect with coworkers, catch up on the latest gossip, and bond over a shared love for coffee's rich, smooth taste.

Sometimes, I even schedule coffee breaks with coworkers, using them as an opportunity to step away from my desk, stretch my legs, and recharge my batteries. It's a way to break up the monotony of the workday and enjoy a few moments of relaxation with friends.

In the end, my love of coffee at work is about more than just the beverage itself. It's about the routine, comfort, and camaraderie it brings. And, as I take my last sip of the day, I know that tomorrow will bring another opportunity to enjoy my beloved coffee at work

CHAPTER 10: COFFEE AND SOCIALIZING

Ah, coffee and socializing – the scrumptious combination. For me, there's nothing quite like the rich aroma of freshly brewed coffee mixed with laughter and lively conversation. It's like a warm blanket on a cold day, wrapping me up in comfort and joy.

I love nothing more than meeting up with friends, family, or coworkers over a cup of coffee. It's a chance to catch up, share stories, and connect deeper. Whether it's a quick coffee break during a busy day or a leisurely afternoon spent in a cozy cafe, coffee and socializing come hand in hand.

One of my favorite ways to enjoy coffee and socializing is by hosting a coffee get-together at my home. I'll brew up a pot of coffee, set out a selection of pastries and snacks, and invite friends over for a cozy afternoon of conversation and relaxation.

It's a chance to slow down and savor the moment, to appreciate the simple pleasures of life.

But coffee and socializing isn't just about relaxing at home. It's also about exploring different places and trying out different things. I love visiting new cafes, coffee shops, and coffee festivals, immersing myself in coffee culture. It's a chance to discover bursting flavors, learn about coffee history, and connect with like-minded individuals.

And, let's not forget about coffee's social aspect. Whether it's a quick chat with a coworker over a cup of coffee or a more formal meeting with clients, coffee brings people together. It's a chance to break down barriers, find common ground, and build relationships that last a lifetime.

But, my love for coffee and socializing isn't just about the taste and the connections. It's also about memories. Some of my favorite moments in life have been spent sipping coffee with loved ones, sharing stories, and laughing until our sides ache. It's these moments that I cherish, moments that bring meaning and joy to my life.

So, whether I'm hosting a coffee get-together at home, exploring nearby coffee shops and cafes, or simply chatting with friends and coworkers over a cup of coffee, I know I'm experiencing something special. Something that connects me to the world around me, that brings me joy and comfort, and that creates memories that last a lifetime. Coffee and socializing – it's the perfect combination.

PART 4

BEYOND THE CUP

CHAPTER 11: COFFEE AND HEALTH

As a self-proclaimed coffee aficionado, I've always been fascinated by the beverage that is a staple in my daily routine. Beyond the cup, coffee has a rich history and is associated with various health benefits, which I recently discovered on my exploration journey. Let me take you on an adventure through the world of "Coffee and Health," where we'll delve into scientific research, dispel some myths, and uncover some surprising truths about how coffee can impact our well-being.

My curiosity about coffee and its effects on health was piqued when I stumbled upon a headline that proclaimed "Coffee: A Magical Elixir for Health!" Intrigued, I delved deeper into the topic, eager to learn more about the potential benefits of my beloved beverage. As I delved into research, I realized that coffee was more to coffee than just its invigorating taste and aroma.

I started my journey by exploring the scientific literature on the topic. To my surprise, I discovered that coffee is packed with powerful antioxidants that can fight inflammation and reduce the risk of chronic diseases such as heart disease, type 2 diabetes, and even some types of cancer. These antioxidants, including chlorogenic acid and polyphenols, are naturally occurring compounds found in coffee beans. They have been shown to have anti-inflammatory properties and can protect our bodies from harmful free radicals.

As I continued my research, I was delighted to find out that coffee has been associated with improved cognitive function and a reduced risk of neurological diseases such as Parkinson's and Alzheimer's. Studies have shown that coffee enhances cognitive performance, including memory, attention, and alertness. This is thanks to its caffeine content, which stimulates the central nervous system.

In addition to its potential cognitive benefits, I also discovered that coffee could be a potent ally in our battle against excess weight. Caffeine boosts metabolism and increases fat oxidation, helping with weight loss and weight management. Moreover, coffee can also suppress appetites, helping us feel fuller for longer and potentially reducing our calorie intake. Of course, it's worthwhile to note that adding excessive amounts of cream, sugar, and other high-calorie additives to coffee can negate these potential benefits, so it's wise to enjoy it in moderation and with minimal added extras.

On my quest for knowledge, I also came across some myths and misconceptions about coffee and health that needed to be addressed. One common myth is that coffee causes dehydration. However, research has shown that moderate coffee consumption does not have a dehydrating effect on the body, as the diuretic effect of caffeine is mild and can be offset by coffee's water content. In fact, coffee can contribute to our daily fluid intake, just like any other beverage.

Another myth I encountered was the belief that coffee could lead to osteoporosis or weaken bones. However, studies have shown that moderate coffee consumption does not significantly increase bone loss or fracture risk. In fact, some research suggests coffee may even protect bone health. This is possibly due to its high mineral content, including magnesium and calcium.

As my exploration journey continued, I also learned about some of the potential downsides of excessive coffee consumption.

Too much caffeine can lead to unwanted side effects such as nervousness, anxiety, insomnia, and even addiction in some cases. It's essential to know our individual caffeine tolerance and consume coffee in moderation. This is particularly true when we are sensitive to its effects or have pre-existing health conditions that may be exacerbated by excessive caffeine intake.

In addition, coffee can also stain our teeth and cause unsanitary breath due to its acidity and dark pigments. However, these cosmetic concerns can be mitigated with regular dental hygiene practices such as brushing, flossing, and rinsing after

CHAPTER 12: THE DARK SIDE OF COFFEE

As I continued my journey of exploring the world of coffee and its impact on health, I stumbled upon a lesser-known subtopic that intrigued me: "The Dark Side of Coffee." While coffee has been associated with numerous health benefits, there are also some potential downsides to be aware of, and I was eager to dig deeper into this aspect of my beloved beverage.

One of the first issues I discovered in my research was the potential negative impact of excessive caffeine consumption. As a natural stimulant, caffeine can have both positive and negative effects on our bodies. While moderate caffeine intake has been linked to improved cognitive function, increased alertness, and enhanced physical performance, excessive caffeine consumption can lead to a variety of issues.

One of the most common side effects of too much caffeine is nervousness and anxiety. As a central nervous system stimulant, caffeine increases heart rate, blood pressure, and trigger stress hormones. This leads to jitteriness and unease. Additionally, excessive caffeine intake can disrupt sleep patterns, leading to insomnia or poor sleep quality, which can affect our overall health and well-being.

Another potential downside of coffee is its impact on the digestive system. Coffee is a known gastrointestinal irritant and can cause gastrointestinal discomfort for some people, such as acid reflux, indigestion, and stomach ulcers. This is especially true for individuals who are prone to these conditions or have pre-existing intestinal issues. It's critical to listen to our bodies and know how coffee affects our digestive system. We should consider reducing consumption or switching to a less acidic coffee variety if necessary.

Furthermore, coffee can also affect our oral health. As a dark-colored beverage, coffee can stain our teeth over time, leading to a less-than-desirable appearance. Coffee's high acidity can also erode tooth enamel, leading to tooth sensitivity and dental issues. Regular dental care practices such as brushing, flossing, and rinsing can mitigate these effects. However, it's essential to know the potential impact of coffee on our oral health.

Another concern associated with coffee is its potential for addiction and withdrawal symptoms. Regular coffee consumption can lead to dependence on caffeine. Sudden cessation or reduction of caffeine intake can result in withdrawal symptoms such as headaches, irritability, and fatigue. It's imperative to be mindful of our caffeine consumption and consider gradually reducing our intake if we wish to cut back on coffee. This is to avoid withdrawal effects.

In addition to the potential negative effects on our health, coffee production also has ethical and environmental considerations. Coffee is a globally traded commodity, and the industry has faced issues such as labor exploitation, unfair wages for coffee farmers, deforestation, and habitat destruction. It's worthwhile to know the social and environmental impacts of coffee production. It's important to support ethical and sustainable coffee practices whenever possible, such as buying Fair Trade or Rainforest Alliance certified coffee.

In conclusion, while coffee has been associated with various health benefits, it's critical to know the potential dark side of coffee. Excessive caffeine consumption can cause nervousness, anxiety, disrupted sleep, and gastrointestinal discomfort. Coffee can also have negative impacts on oral health, and it's wise to practice effective dental hygiene. Additionally, coffee production has ethical and environmental considerations that need to be addressed. As with any food or beverage, moderation and mindfulness are key, and it's key to listen to our bodies and make informed choices when it comes to coffee consumption. By being aware of both the positive and negative aspects of coffee, we can enjoy our favorite beverage while taking care of our health and the environment. So, let's raise a cup to a balanced and mindful coffee approach! Cheers!

CHAPTER 13: THE FUTURE OF COFFEE

As I delved into my research on coffee, I couldn't help but wonder what the future of this beloved beverage held. With advancements in technology, changing consumer preferences, and evolving environmental concerns, I was excited to imagine how coffee might look in the years to come.

It was a bright and sunny morning as I walked into my favorite coffee shop, eagerly anticipating my morning brew. As I approached the counter, I noticed something different - there was an entirely different machine behind the barista, unlike any coffee maker I had seen before. The barista greeted me with a smile and explained that it was the latest coffee brewing innovation called the "CoffeeBot 3000." Intrigued, I asked for more information.

The barista explained that the CoffeeBot 3000 was a state-of-the -art coffee brewing machine that used artificial intelligence to analyze individual taste preferences and brew the right cup of coffee tailored to each customer's liking. It had a built-in sensor that detected the exact brewing time, water temperature, and coffee-to-water ratio needed to create the ideal cup of coffee for each person. I was amazed by the precision and customization this machine offered, and I couldn't wait to try it out.

As I sipped on my perfectly brewed cup of coffee, I couldn't help but wonder about coffee production's environmental impact. I had heard about the challenges of deforestation, habitat destruction, and fair labor practices in the coffee industry. I was curious about how things had changed. I decided to dig some more.

To my delight, I discovered that coffee's future was indeed greener and more sustainable. Coffee farmers adopted innovative practices such as agroforestry, where coffee was cultivated alongside other crops, and shade-grown coffee, which preserved natural habitats for birds and wildlife. There was a growing awareness of fair trade practices, and consumers demanded ethically sourced coffee. Additionally, advancements in technology enabled more efficient and environmentally friendly coffee processing methods, such as using renewable energy sources and reducing water consumption.

As I continued to explore the future of coffee, I also came across some unique and exciting trends in coffee consumption. Virtual reality coffee tasting experiences gained popularity. This allowed coffee lovers to virtually travel to coffee farms and learn about coffee beans' origin and processing. 3D-printed latte art became the creative expression of baristas, with intricate designs and patterns almost too aesthetically pleasing to drink. Coffee-infused foods and beverages also took the culinary world by storm, with coffee-flavored ice cream, pastries, and cocktails becoming hits among foodies.

Another intriguing development in coffee's future was the rise of "smart" coffee cups. These cups were embedded with sensors that detected the coffee's temperature, freshness, and flavor profile. They could also connect to a smartphone app, allowing users to track coffee consumption, customize brewing settings, and order coffee for delivery. It was a seamless blend of technology and coffee, making coffee drinking even more convenient and personalized.

As I savored my last coffee sip, I couldn't help but reflect on how much the coffee landscape had evolved over the years. From advanced brewing technologies to sustainable farming practices, and from virtual reality tastings to smart coffee cups, the future of coffee is indeed a world of innovation, sustainability, and customization. I was excited to see what other exciting developments were in store for coffee, and I couldn't wait to embark on more coffee adventures in the future.

With a contented smile, I left the coffee shop, looking forward to the next chapter in coffee's ever-evolving saga. As I walked down the street, I couldn't help but be grateful for the joy coffee brought

CONCLUSION

A NEVER-ENDING AFFAIR WITH COFFEE

As I drink my steaming cup of coffee, the rich aroma envelops me, bringing back memories of my lifelong love affair with this enchanting elixir. Coffee has been my constant companion, through thick and thin, a loyal confidante that has never let me down. My coffee journey started long ago.

Over the years, my love for coffee grew deeper. It became more than just a beverage; it became a ritual, a moment of solace in life's chaos. From late-night study sessions in college to early morning meetings at work, coffee always provided me with the much-needed energy and comfort. It was my trusted ally during all-nighters, my partner during brainstorming sessions, and my companion during long conversations with friends and loved ones.

But my relationship with coffee transcended beyond its practical benefits. It became a canvas for my imagination, a muse for my creativity. I often lost myself in reverie as I sipped my coffee, imagining far-off lands and embarking on thrilling adventures. Coffee fueled my dreams and inspired me to chase them with gusto.

One particular memory stands out in my mind. I was sitting in a quaint coffee shop in Paris, savoring a cup of freshly brewed French press coffee. The aroma was a symphony of fragrances - hints of chocolate, caramel, and citrus mingled together, creating a sensory experience unlike any other. As I closed my eyes and took a sip, I was transported to Paris' cobbled streets, with the Eiffel Tower standing majestically in the distance. It was as if coffee could teleport me to another world, igniting my wanderlust and filling me with wonder.

But my love affair with coffee wasn't limited to drinking it. I also enjoyed coffee-making, experimenting with different brewing methods, and perfecting my latte art skills. The hissing of the espresso machine, the gentle pour-over of hot water, and the frothing of milk became a symphony of sounds that brought joy to my heart. It was a creative outlet that allowed me to express myself and share my passion for coffee with others.

As I reflect on my never-ending coffee relationship, I am filled with gratitude for the memories and experiences it has brought into my life. It has been more than just a beverage; it has been a source of comfort, inspiration, and adventure. From that first sip as a child to the countless cups I've enjoyed in various corners of the world, coffee has been a constant companion. It has accompanied me through life's ups and downs.

In conclusion, my love affair with coffee will continue to thrive, as I embark on adventurous adventures and create new memories. Coffee has become a part of my identity, a cherished ritual that brings joy to my everyday life. Its alluring aroma, complex flavors, and rich history continue to fascinate me, keeping my obsession with coffee burning bright. With each cup, I am reminded of the magical power of this humble beverage and the endless possibilities it holds. Cheers to a lifetime of endless love and appreciation for coffee! Long live my eternal romance with the brew that captures my heart and awaken my senses. Here's to many more delightful cups of coffee.

EPILOGUE

A PERFECT CUP OF COFFEE

As I sat down at my favorite coffee shop, eagerly anticipating my first sip of the day, I couldn't help but chuckle at the thought of my quest for the " optimum " cup of coffee. You see, despite my years of experience as a coffee aficionado, I still find myself on a never-ending journey to discover the elusive " exceptional " cup of coffee.

As I sipped the steaming hot brew, I couldn't help but wonder - what makes a cup of coffee truly delicious? Is it the type of beans, the brewing method, or the ratio of water to coffee? Or is it just the barista's magical touch that makes all the difference?

I pondered these questions as I struggled to suppress a laugh. I've tried it all - from fancy pour-over gadgets to complicated espresso machines that look like they belong on a spaceship. I've experimented with various brewing techniques, temperatures, and brewing times, all in pursuit of that mythical " ideal " cup of coffee. I've even tried whispering sweet nothings to my coffee beans, hoping to enhance the flavor. But alas, no matter how hard I fought, perfection remained elusive.

I couldn't help but laugh at my own obsession for the perfect cup of coffee. Was it really necessary to obsess over every granular detail, or should I just sit back, relax, and enjoy my coffee without overthinking it? I realized that my pursuit of perfection had become comical, and perhaps it was time to let go of my coffee perfectionionism and simply enjoy the experience.

As I sipped my coffee, I couldn't help but notice the absurdity of it all. I mean, how many times have I asked myself questions like, "Is this the perfect water-to-coffee ratio?" or "Did I grind the beans to the exact right coarseness?" It was almost as if I was trying to solve a complex mathematical equation with every sip?

I chuckled as I looked around the coffee shop and wondered how many other fellow coffee lovers were on a similar quest for coffee perfection. Were they meticulously measuring their coffee grounds with a scale? Were they timing their brews to the second? Or were they simply enjoying their coffee without fuss?

As I finished my coffee and got up to leave, I realized that the pursuit of the ideally appointed cup of coffee was never-ending. Perhaps that was part of the fun. It was the journey, the experimentation, and the occasional coffee mishaps that made it all so entertaining. After all, life would be boring without adventure, even brewing a cup of coffee.

So, as I walked out of the coffee shop with a smile on my face, I left behind my quest for perfection. Instead, I embraced the joy of enjoying a cup of coffee, flaws and all. I realized that the happiest cup of coffee was not about perfection, but about savoring the moment. I added a dash of humor along the way.

So, dear reader, I leave you with these questions to ponder over your next cup of coffee: Is there such a thing as the perfect cup of coffee? Or is perfection part of the fun? Perhaps the real joy of coffee lies not in perfection, but in the quirks, surprises, and laughter that comes with each cup. Cheers to embracing imperfections and enjoying coffee appreciation's hilarious journey! Keep brewing, experimenting, and laughing, and may your coffee always smile. Cheers! And remember, it's just coffee, not rocket science!